Your body is your most essential piece of dive equipment.
Are you maintaining it as well as the rest of your gear?

Adams & Adams
Fit for SCUBA

a strength and conditioning handbook

Jessica B. Adams, M.S.
and
Jaime B. Adams, M.S.

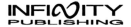
INFINITY
PUBLISHING

Copyright © 2006 by Jessica B. Adams and Jaime B. Adams

ISBN 978-0-7414-3111-0

Published by:

INFINITY
PUBLISHING

INFINITY PUBLISHING

Toll-free (877) BUY BOOK
Local Phone (610) 941-9999
Fax (610) 941-9959
Info@buybooksontheweb.com
www.buybooksontheweb.com

Printed in the United States of America
Published November 2012

CREDITS

Editors: Neal Pollock, Janet Hayes-DelTufo, Liz Marmesh, Mary Hayes-Macaluso, Tom Macaluso, and Wesley Smith

Photography: Jessica Adams, Jaime Adams, Dru Adams, Philip Brossard, Mary Hayes-Macaluso, and the Wellness Center at Broward Community College

Cover Design: Jessica Adams, Jaime Adams, and Donner Valle

DEDICATION

This book is dedicated to everyone working to improve dive safety and to all those interested in a healthy pursuit, respect, and appreciation of our underwater world.

ACKNOWLEDGMENTS

We would like to thank everyone that has supported this project! Your input was a vital part to the success of *Fit for SCUBA*.

We are especially grateful to our families for their continuous support of our crazy dreams.

TABLE OF CONTENTS

PREFACE

Wetsuit manufacturers are creating bigger and BIGGER sizes each year to accommodate divers. Out-of-shape divers are getting in the water and at times getting into trouble. Unfortunately, we are seeing an increasing number of unfit divers in emergency rooms and morgues around the world. No! Scuba diving is not becoming a more dangerous activity. Divers are concerned with safety: we have buddies, follow dive plans, keep dive logs, and complete routine maintenance of our gear. However, many of us neglect the most vital piece of equipment…our bodies.

Congratulations! With this manual, you now have the tools to become a safer, more fit diver. By applying these simple instructions and following the illustrations in this manual, you will improve your fitness level, regardless of your current level of fitness. Deciding to participate in a fitness program may be the best decision that you can make to improve the quality of your diving experience. Now all you have to do is follow through on your plan. Furthermore, you will see drastic improvements in your overall quality of life.

True, this is a challenging endeavor, but as a trained scuba diver, you already possess many of the attributes necessary for success. You are probably the type of person who enjoys new challenges. You have already successfully applied training, planning, and focus to meet the demands of your certification course(s). If you apply these skills to your fitness program, your fitness level is certain to improve over time. Plan your workout and exercise according to your plan. As a diver, you are probably already quite adept at making a plan, following through, and maintaining accurate records of your experiences. These attributes will help you to implement a successful fitness program.

Your fitness program must be a regular part of your life, in order to maintain these improvements. It should be just as much a part of your regular routine as taking a shower and brushing your teeth. The best program for you is one that you will realistically maintain for years to come. For this reason, we have provided workouts for the home as well as in the gym. You will find activities suitable for every environment. This program should be a part of your routine, no matter where you are. There are no excuses for not making a commitment to your body and yourself. After all, you deserve it.

Although you would probably like to be immersed in water every day, the reality is that most of you are forced to be weekend warriors due to the commitments of daily life. Unfortunately, this lifestyle may cause the typical recreational scuba diver to only be active on weekends or dive vacations. This type of exercise schedule results in minimal training and may lead to injuries. It also does not prepare you for the unexpected challenges that you may encounter during your dive. An increased level of comfort in the water will create a more enjoyable scuba experience as well as an increased energy level for your dive vacation both in and out of the water.

Due to common misconceptions, scuba diving has been highly ignored by the fitness industry. As you know, dive gear alone places an additional load on the body. The physical demands of entries and exits must also be considered. Above all, scuba divers must always be physically and mentally prepared for challenging conditions that may arise in this dynamic underwater world. As you know, almost every diver has a story about a difficult exit from the water or a challenging current.

A proper fitness program will prepare you to more effectively deal with the challenges that you may encounter during your dive. Improved muscular strength will minimize the stress of pre- and post-dive equipment handling. Entries and exits will also be completed with greater ease. Increased muscular and cardiovascular efficiency may improve comfort and confidence during your dive. Improved strength, flexibility, and balance will add comfort to maneuvering around a rocking boat, particularly when you are wearing your gear. You and your dive buddy will benefit from increased confidence in personal capabilities, allowing a more relaxing and enjoyable underwater experience. You will also experience a boost in your overall energy level! Some additional benefits of exercise include:

- Improved cardiovascular health
- Weight control

- Lower blood lipids

- Decreased blood pressure

- Increased bone density

- Psychological benefits

Make the health of your body one of the essential commitments in your life. For a more relaxed scuba diving experience, you will benefit from a conditioning program, which improves flexibility, strength, endurance, and balance. Your body is a unique machine that responds directly to training. It is time to start training your body. This is the only body that you will ever get, so take care of it!

This fitness program has been developed with you, the scuba diver, in mind. Strength is developed in areas of the body that are utilized during your dive. If you follow the simple guidelines of this book, you will have the knowledge to create a fitness program that will work for you. No single fitness program exists that will be successful for each of you. Our goal is to give you the tools to create a program that will fit *your* lifestyle and yield the results that you need. Remember, a successful fitness program takes planning as well as commitment…just like a successful dive!

CHAPTER 1

Introduction

This is your body; therefore, it is your responsibility to be proactive in preparation for a safe and exciting scuba-diving experience. Provided you are physically fit, no upper age limit exists for scuba diving. Fortunately, diving can be a lifelong activity if you maintain the proper level of fitness. Our goal is to give you the knowledge to create a program that will allow scuba diving to be a part of your life for many decades to come. We want you to retire from work, not from diving, so we must maintain a level of fitness that allows us to safely appreciate the underwater world for years to come. It is never too late to get in shape!

These workouts will become a part of your regular weekly routine. Three components of your program are vital to long-term success. First, you must develop a program that is enjoyable. This means working out with a buddy, or perhaps you are the type of person that prefers independently working out. Whatever your preference, create an environment that appeals to you. Second, your exercise routine must realistically fit into your schedule. If you cannot fit in an hour at a time, try to break up your routine into smaller, more frequent blocks of time. Finally, hold yourself accountable for completing your workouts by keeping a logbook or reporting to a friend. If you follow these simple guidelines, you will find it easier to maintain your program for the long haul. Many individuals start a fitness program "gung ho" and fade out. Pace yourself; this is a marathon, not a sprint.

For your safety, there are a few rules of thumb when training. Always execute proper form during all exercises. This should be easy for you if you focus on the simple instructions and illustrations provided in this text. For the best results, form is always a priority over weight. Proper technique also reduces incidence of injury. Stop immediately if you experience breathlessness, dizziness, or pain. If you injure yourself, you may have to take days or weeks to recover. This leads to detraining. Safety always takes priority. Remember, there should be no training within 12 hours of diving and all training should be preceded and followed with proper hydration. But above all, remember to have fun!

Everyone should have a clean bill of health from his or her yearly physical exam prior to beginning an exercise program. As with all new activities, if you have any of the following risk factors, make sure that you consult your physician before beginning an exercise program.

- Over the age of 35
- Hypertension
- High cholesterol
- High triglycerides
- Diabetes
- Prior health complications
- Smoker
- Heart trouble
- Fainting
- Pregnant
- Joint problems

Keep in mind that a sedentary lifestyle (inactivity) is also a risk factor for cardiovascular disease.

Avoid strenuous exercise within 24 hours of diving.

CHAPTER 2

Developing Your Program

A successful training program is one that will allow you to make a long-term commitment to yourself. Positive results take commitment, time, and patience. Fortunately, you have already developed these attributes during your scuba-certification training. Remember, you are not only improving your scuba experience, but also your overall quality of life.

In order to develop a successful program, you must first answer a few questions realistically and honestly.

1. Why am I starting an exercise program?
2. Where will I implement my training? (HOME vs. GYM)
3. How many days per week will I exercise?
4. How much time can I commit per session?

Make a record of your responses as well as your training program. Training logs are available in Appendix I of this text. Record the time of day and how you feel along with any other relevant information. It is also important to document how hard you are working; you may use the rate of perceived exertion chart in chapter 12 of this text. Terms such as *light, somewhat hard, hard*, or *very hard* are also effective for documenting intensity levels. Keep a logbook just as you do for your dives. This is for your future reference and planning. Your exercise log serves the same purpose as your dive log. An accurate logbook will help you to identify the causes of positive as well as negative results. This will aid in modification of your program, so you can successfully achieve the results that will improve your scuba experiences.

The response to question #1 is going to be your long-term goal. This could be your next dive vacation, next year, or even five years down the road. Once you have an attainable long-term goal, set a series of short-term goals to get you there. Where do you realistically see yourself in three months, two months, one month, two weeks, and one week? Then make a plan for yourself. This plan should consist of a series of specific short-term goals to reach your long-term goal set in response to our first question. An example of a short-term weekly goal may be to complete one set of each exercise. Make sure your goals are specific and realistically within reach. If not, we all have a tendency to become discouraged. The key to success is taking baby steps toward your goals and avoiding injury. This is not a quick fix, but rather a lifelong project.

In the chapters to follow, exercises that can be implemented at home as well as in the gym are included. You should commit a minimum of three days per week and 30 minutes per session. It does not matter if your workouts are done at home or in the gym as long as you complete them. If you happen to miss a workout, simply make it up. This is a lifelong program.

When developing your program, start at a low intensity and gradually increase your weights, sets, and repetitions as your body allows. Weight is the amount you lift through a single range of motion. Repetitions are the number of times that you go through a given range of motion before taking a break. Sets are the number of groups of repetitions that you complete for a given exercise. For example, you may complete one set of ten repetitions of a bench press given a weight of 75 pounds.

A good starting point is one set of ten repetitions. This is because your initial strength gains are predominantly neurological rather than physiological. At this point, your brain is learning how to send the most efficient signals to your muscles to perform a new exercise. Proper form is vital at this time in your programming. After about two weeks, you can increase to two sets of ten repetitions. By week three, you should increase to three sets of ten repetitions. From there, you can gradually increase your repetitions to 12, then 15. Once you have successfully achieved three sets of 15 repetitions of a given weight, it is time to increase the weight and drop your sets back down to ten repetitions. Repeat this process throughout your program. An indication that you are lifting the proper weight is that the final repetition of the final set should be very hard. Ideally, you should not have enough energy remaining to complete another repetition.

Your program should address strength training, cardiovascular training, and flexibility training. These components of fitness will complement one another throughout your dive, as well as your daily life. We will also integrate a component of balance so that you are more comfortable maneuvering on those rough days out on the boat. Improvements in both strength and balance will make donning gear and entering the water more comfortable.

We have outlined some of the muscles used during common dive-related activities so that you can tailor a program to meet your diving needs.

Ventral Musculature

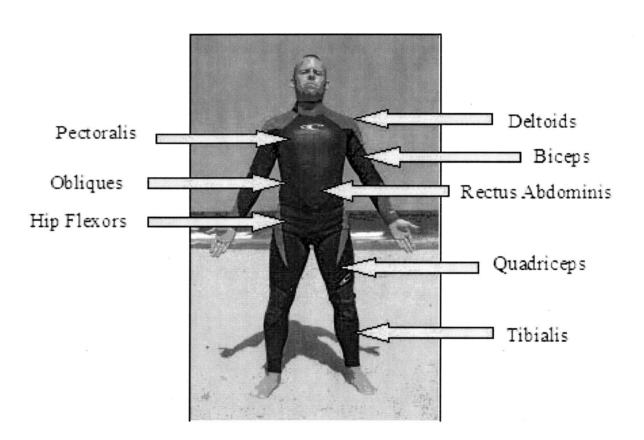

Pectoralis

Obliques

Hip Flexors

Deltoids

Biceps

Rectus Abdominis

Quadriceps

Tibialis

Dorsal Musculature

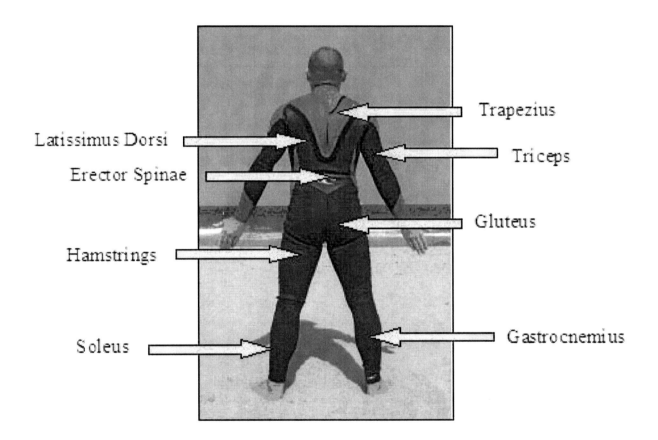

Trapezius

Latissimus Dorsi

Triceps

Erector Spinae

Gluteus

Hamstrings

Soleus

Gastrocnemius

Diving Activities	Muscles
Carrying Gear	Back – latissimus dorsi, trapezius Shoulders – deltoids Legs – quadriceps, gluteus
Stepping On/Off Boat	Legs – quadriceps, hamstrings, gastrocnemius, soleus Back – erector spinae
Walking with Gear (beach)	Legs – quadriceps, hamstrings, gastrocnemius, soleus Back – erector spinae
Getting Up from Bench with Gear On	Legs – quadriceps, hamstrings, gluteus, hip flexors, gastrocnemius, soleus Back – erector spinae Arms – triceps
Finning (kicking)	Hips – flexors, extensors Legs – gluteus, quadriceps, hamstrings, gastrocnemius, soleus, tibialis
Climbing Up the Ladder	Back – latissimus dorsi, trapezius, Shoulders – deltoids

We have also listed the exercises available throughout the text according to muscle group. This way you can easily plan out the exercises that you would like to integrate into your program.

BODY PART	GYM	HOME
Legs	Squat Leg Press Leg Extension Leg Curl Standing Calf Raise	Chair/Box Squat Body Squat Stationary Lunge Stability Ball Leg Curl Standing Calf Raise
Chest	Bench Press Pec Deck	Pushup Dumbbell Press Dumbbell Fly
Shoulders	Military Shoulder Press	Shoulder Press Front/Lateral Shoulder Raises
Upper Back	Lat Pull Down Seated Row	Upright Row Bent Over Row
Lower Back	Roman Chair	Back Extensions Quadruped Arm and Leg Raise
Abs	Progression Back Press Crunches Twisting Crunch Ball Crunch	Progression Back Press Crunch Twisting Crunch Ball Crunch
Triceps	Dip Triceps Push Down	Chair Dip Triceps Kickback
Biceps	Preacher Curl	Biceps Curl

Remember, when working on strength training, proper form always takes priority over the amount of weight lifted. Make sure that you begin all standing exercises in an athletic stance (see pg. 30), which emphasizes proper body position and form. Your feet are shoulder width apart; toes are pointed slightly outward; knees are slightly bent; shoulders and buttocks are back in the athletic stance. An athletic stance is illustrated in chapter 5. When performing the exercises, do not rest the weights in between repetitions. This will allow constant tension to be placed on the muscle until the set is complete.

Now that you have the basics, it is time to select your exercises. You may select any number of exercises for each muscle group. The exercises for specific muscle groups are identified at the beginning of each chapter. It is important that you balance your workout. Balancing means that you include an equal number of exercises, sets, and repetitions for opposing muscle groups. Opposing muscle groups include:

Chest ↔ Upper Back

Abdominals ↔ Lower Back

Quadriceps ↔ Hamstrings

Biceps ↔ Triceps

You may select any exercises, provided your workout is balanced. When planning your program, an additional consideration is recovery time. Each muscle group needs a 24-48 hour rest period in between workouts for recovery.

This text has provided samples of three- and four-day workouts in Appendix II. These are only guidelines. Remember, the best program for you is one you will maintain for years to come. In order to make this a lifelong program, start with lightweight and simple movements. Also make sure that you progress slowly. As you acclimate and become stronger, increase the weight to continue to challenge your muscles. You should be able to perform the appropriate number of repetitions no more and no less. If you are able to do many extra repetitions, it is an indication to use a higher weight. If you cannot complete your repetitions, you may want to decrease the weight to finish your set. Some days are better than others, so adjusting the weight is appropriate. These methods of training will maximize your long-term benefits.

CHAPTER 3

Warm-up and Cool-down

The warm-up is an essential part of your exercise routine. Cold muscles do not possess an effective range of motion to exercise without risk of injury. In addition, warm muscles aid in a quality workout. An effective warm-up can increase the amount of force production during your workout. There are numerous variations of warming up your muscles. However, the primary principle of all variations is to elevate the core muscle temperature and maintain that temperature throughout your workout. Hence, the term warm-up. We will address three general concepts behind the warm-up.

The most common type is the general warm-up. This consists of ten to 15 minutes of cardiovascular activity. Cardiovascular activities include, but are not limited to, biking, jogging, stair stepping, and elliptical machines. This is effective in elevating your core body temperature; however, it may not target the specific muscle groups that you are trying to work on a given day. A general warm-up is beneficial if your primary goal is to improve your cardiovascular endurance.

Another type is the specific warm-up. This consists of one to three sets of lightweight repetitions of each exercise that you are going to perform that day. It is important to do enough work to elevate muscle temperature. This is very effective at targeting specific muscle groups. A specific warm-up is beneficial if your primary goal is increasing muscular strength. This will make carrying tanks and gear easier for you. Exits from the water will be executed with greater ease.

The third type that we will address is the functional warm-up. This consists of strengthening commonly weak muscle groups. Functional warm-ups include a combination of abdominal and lower back exercises, such as those found in chapters 10 and 11. It is important to minimize time between different exercises to maintain an overall elevated temperature. A functional warm-up is useful when your primary goal is strengthening core musculature and improving balance. This will aid in maneuvering around a rocking boat, donning gear, and entering the water. This type of warm-up is of great value to individuals prone to lower back pain.

Your cooldown is just as important as your warm-up. If you stop immediately after strenuous exercise, you are placing an increased load on your heart. Additionally, missing a cooldown can lead to light-headedness. The best way to minimize post exercise soreness is to complete an active recovery. An active recovery consists of a low level of physical activity followed by your flexibility exercise routine. A few activities that can be included in your cooldown are light jogging, cycling, and walking. This will decrease the post-exercise load on your heart. It will also decrease muscle soreness. An additional benefit is improved flexibility due to the elevated core muscle temperature during your stretching routine. This is a direct benefit of stretching after exercise.

CHAPTER 4

Flexibility

Flexibility is a key component of your fitness program for diving. With a good range of motion, putting on gear, entries, and exits will be executed with greater ease. Flexibility also aids in maneuvering around a rocking boat without falling. An increased range of motion also minimizes lower back pain. If flexibility is not addressed during your workout, your range of motion can actually decrease. This is due to the increased muscle mass acquired during training. However, a good flexibility routine properly integrated into your workout will enhance your overall range of motion.

Flexibility training must occur when the body temperature is elevated. It is important to gradually increase the range of a stretch and hold it for between 30 and 90 seconds. Then take a breath, exhale, and attempt to increase the stretch. This new position should also be held for a minimum of 30 seconds. Although bouncing may appear to increase your range of motion, this can actually tear your muscle fibers. This may ultimately decrease your range of motion. All movements should be smooth and controlled.

Stretch	Muscles	Scuba Applications
Doorway Stretch	Pectoralis	
Pretzel	Erector Spinae Obliques	• Putting on BCD
Lat Stretch	Latissimus dorsi	• Putting on fins
Cross Body Stretch	Latissimus dorsi	
Arm Circles	Deltoids	• Reaching for ladder/tag lines
Behind the Neck	Triceps	• Arm overhead on ascents
Modified Hurdler	Hamstrings	
Seated Hamstrings	Hamstrings	• Reaching hoses/tank valves
Stair Stretch	Gastrocnemius Soleus	• Putting on wetsuits
Wall Push	Gastrocnemius Soleus	• Climbing ladders
Lying / Standing Quadriceps Stretch	Quadriceps	• "Duck Walk" with fins
Abdominal Stretch	Abdominals	

Hint

A typical commercial lasts between 30 and 60 seconds, which just happens to be the duration for holding a stretch. If you complete one stretching exercise per commercial during your favorite television show, your flexibility training can be completed by the end of the show.

CHEST

Doorway Stretch

Stand in a doorway and place one arm against the wall. Slightly turn the upper body away from the wall.

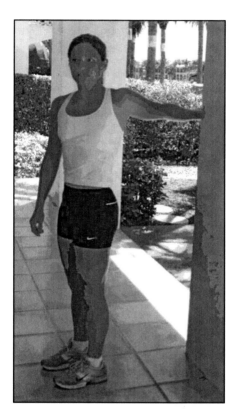

Scuba Application

Flexibility in your pectoral area will make putting on those BCDs and wetsuits much easier.

LOWER BACK

Pretzel

Begin by sitting on the floor with legs fully extended. Bend one leg at the knee and cross it over the other. Place the foot just outside the knee of the extended leg. Cross the body with the opposite arm and place the elbow on the inside of the opposite knee. Turn the shoulders and torso away from the knee. This will stretch the lower back.

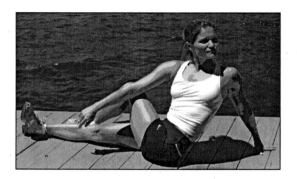 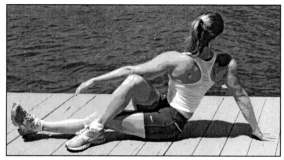

Scuba Application

This will make donning gear more comfortable, especially those fins. An increased range of motion in your lower back will also minimize lower back pain.

UPPER BACK

Lat Stretch

Kneel on the floor. Reach out in front of you with both hands placing your palms down on the floor. Simultaneously lower your chest to the floor and your knees. This will stretch your upper back and shoulders.

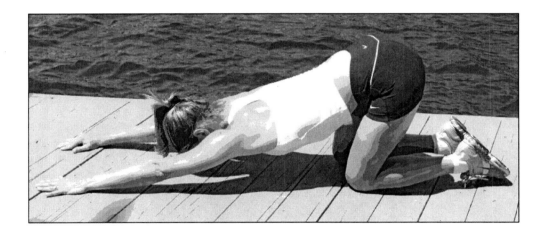

Scuba Application

An increased range of motion in your upper back will make it easier to reach those hoses, just in case you lose your regulator. This is of particular importance to technical divers who need to reach their tank valves.

UPPER BACK

Cross Body Stretch

Extend one arm across the body just below the chin. Reach up with opposite hand and grasp the elbow. Gently pull the arm across the body with the opposite hand.

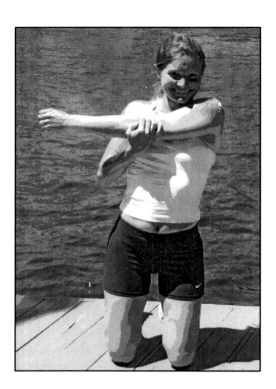

Scuba Application

This will make taking off your wetsuit much easier.

SHOULDERS

Arm Circles

Extend both arms straight out at your sides. Begin with small circles forwards and backwards for 12 repetitions each. Then increase the size of circles for both directions.

Small Circles   **Large Circles**

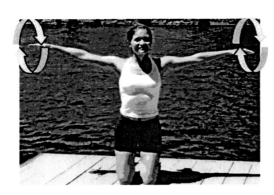
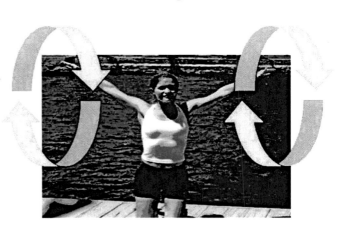

Scuba Applications

A good range of motion in your shoulder joint will allow you to put your hand above your head during ascents. It will also be easier to reach for ladders and tag lines. Remember, you never know when you might need to reach for the railing of a rocking boat.

TRICEPS

Behind the Neck

Extend one arm straight up like you are pointing to the sky. Bend the same arm at the elbow, so the elbow is pointing to the sky. To increase the stretch, lightly pull the elbow toward the back with the opposite hand.

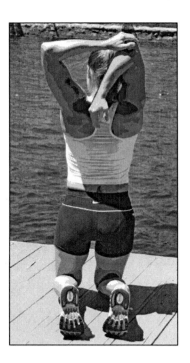

Scuba Application

An increased range of motion in your triceps makes reaching for hoses and tank valves much more comfortable.

HAMSTRINGS

Modified Hurdler

While seated on the floor, extend both feet out in front. Bend one leg and place the sole of the foot just inside the other knee. Reach with both hands together toward the toes of the extended leg.

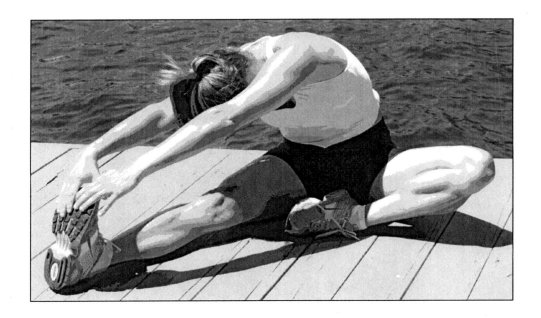

Tip

Keep your head down.

Seated Hamstrings Stretch

A similar stretch can be done while sitting in a chair. Sit toward the edge of a chair to allow one leg to be fully extended. For support, the other leg should be at a 90-degree angle. Reach toward the toes of the extended leg with both hands. Keep the leg as straight as possible to get the best stretch.

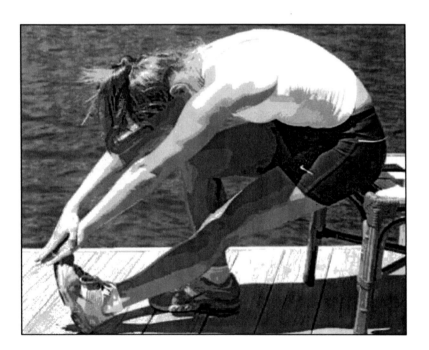

Scuba Application

A good range of motion in your hamstrings will allow you to put on your wetsuit and fins with greater ease.

CALVES

Stair Stretch

Start by standing with the balls of the feet on a step. It probably isn't wise to use the top step. Lower the heels toward the floor. One at a time is best for balance. Bending the knee of the non-stretching leg will help increase the stretch.

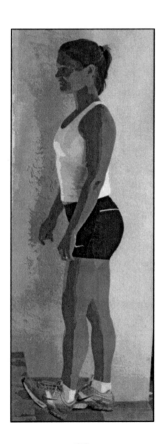

Chair Push

Face a chair or wall with a scissors stance, one foot in front and the other back. Slightly bend the knee of the front leg while the back leg remains straight. Push against the wall slightly with the hands. Concentrate on the legs, bending the front leg, and keeping the heel down on the rear foot will increase the stretch.

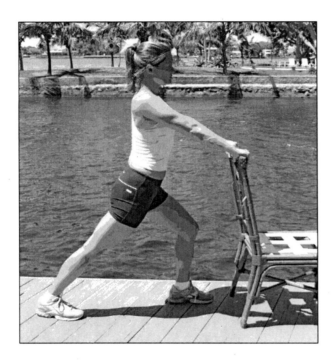

Scuba Application

A good range of motion in your calf will allow you to relieve those nasty calf cramps from finning on your own. You will also notice a marked improvement in your duck walk with fins.

ABDOMINAL STRETCH

***Avoid this stretch if you are prone to lower back pain. ***

Begin by lying on the floor supported by your elbows; you should feel the stretch in your abdominals.

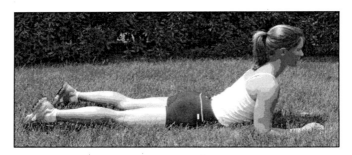

When you no longer feel the stretch, try pressing with your hands. Your hands should be directly underneath your shoulders and press up as far as you can.

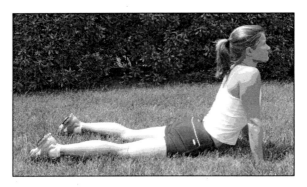

Scuba Application

A good range of motion in your abdominals will make donning gear more comfortable.

QUADRICEPS

Lying Quadriceps Stretch

Begin lying on your side with both legs extended. Extend the bottom arm for support. Bend the upper leg at the knee and bring the heel to the rear. Reach back and grasp the leg at the ankle of the bent knee. To increase the stretch, slowly point the knee backwards while continuing to support the leg at the ankle.

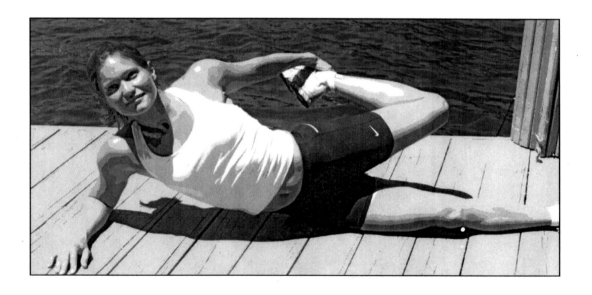

Tip

Pull your leg straight back while pushing forward through your hips.

Standing Quadriceps Stretch

A wall or chair is good to use for support. Bend one knee and bring the heel to the rear. Grasp the leg at the ankle with the knee pointing to the ground. To increase the stretch, push the knee further back. Don't bring the knee to the side because this may increase the stress on the knee. A slight forward body lean may be necessary, so remember the supports. The form is the same as the lying quadriceps stretch, however you are standing.

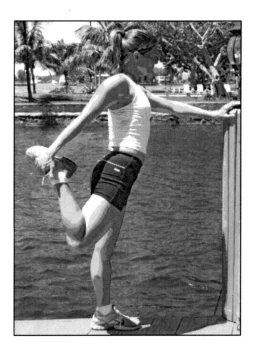

Scuba Application

A good range of motion in your quadriceps will make donning gear more comfortable.

27

CHAPTER 5

General Weight Training Tips

1. Always make sure that you are in control of the weight. The weight should not determine your range of motion. If the weight pulls your body, it could cause tearing of the muscles, tendons, or ligaments. This type of injury may force you to take weeks off of your training routine.

2. Do not rest the weights between repetitions. Maintain tension on the muscle throughout the entire set. This will maximize the stress on your muscle, yielding the greatest improvements in strength.

3. Never bounce; this could cause tearing of your muscles. Movements should always be smooth and controlled to maximize your strength gains while minimizing risk of injury.

4. Never ever hold your breath! You should already be a pro at this one. Holding your breath during a lift causes a spike in blood pressure. This places an excessive load on your heart. Exhale....

5. Always have a spotter when you are attempting a challenging lift. This will allow you to safely push your upper limits.

6. Gradual progression is necessary for fitness improvements without injury.

Simple → Complex

Light Weight → Heavier Weight

Short Duration → Longer Duration

7. Make sure that you are lifting the proper amount of weight. After the final repetition of your last set, the muscle group being worked should be fatigued. At this time, you should not be able to complete another repetition at this weight.

8. Always maintain an athletic stance, chest and buttocks out. This creates the most stable position for vertebral alignment. It will minimize back injuries in addition to isolating particular muscle groups.

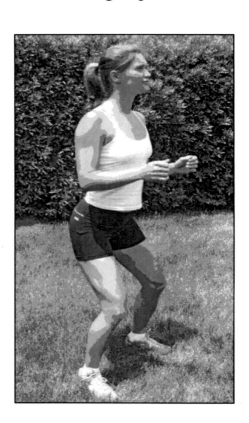

CHAPTER 6

Lower Body Home Exercises

Exercise	Muscles	Scuba Application
Chair/Box Squat	Quadriceps Gluteus Hip Flexors	• Rising from bench • Sitting on bench
Body Squat	Quadriceps Gluteus Hip Flexors	• Walking in gear • Walking in sand
Stationary Lunge	Quadriceps Gluteus Hip Flexors	• Setting gear on bench
Standing Calf Raise	Gastrocnemius Soleus	• Finning
Stability Ball Leg Curl	Hamstrings Gluteus Erector Spinae	• Ascending/Descending ladder

Hint:

The beauty of lower body home exercises is that sets can be completed in time frames as short as two minutes throughout the day at home or in the office. These exercises take little preparation or equipment. Be creative with your routines. If you give yourself short breaks throughout your day to get your blood flowing, you may even be more productive at work.

CHAIR/BOX SQUAT

This is an introduction to the squat. The chair is used for a reference to add comfort to the sitting back motion. It aids in keeping your knees behind your toes and weight on your heels.

Setup

Stand in athletic stance with feet shoulder width apart and toes pointing slightly outward. Keep your shoulders and buttocks back, and stick your chest out. The chair should be approximately one foot behind you.

Exercise

1. Bend your knees, keeping your weight over your heels.
2. You may put your hands forwards for balance.
3. Squat down as close to the chair as you can. Throughout this motion, you should be able to wiggle your toes.
4. Without actually sitting in the chair, press up through your heels returning to standing position.
5. Your head and chest should be up for the complete motion.

Tip

Look straight ahead or slightly toward the sky.

The chair or box squat is just a squat done with the assistance of a chair. The chair is used more for a reference than as an aid. In short, squat to the chair and stand up. Dumbbells can be added to increase resistance. This is just like standing up from a bench on a dive boat. Remember, on the boat, you will be loaded with gear. This is a good starting point.

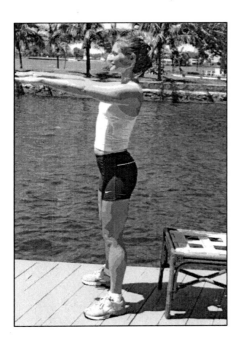 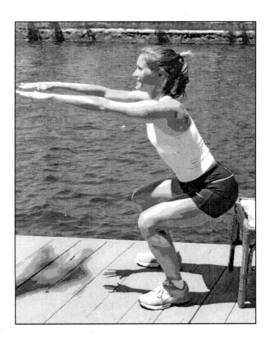

Scuba Application

This will allow you to rise from a bench in full gear with less effort. It will also make climbing that ladder after your dive easier.

Hint

You can squeeze in some of your workout at the office by completing sets throughout your day.

BODY SQUAT

As we stated earlier, the squat is a great exercise for the lower body. The body squat is actually the first step in the progression of weighted squats. This exercise can be done at home with body weight alone. Simply, squat from the standing position, by bending the knees and lowering the hips toward the floor.

Setup

In the standing position, the feet should be slightly wider than shoulder width apart with the toes pointed slightly outward. The back should always be flat. The rear should be emphasized as being out.

Exercise

1. Bend the knees, allowing the (hips) to move toward the floor.

2. Maintain a flat and rigid back.

3. Look forward with the chest out.

4. Knees should be aligned over the feet.

5. Don't let knees go over the toes (leaning forward is not good).

6. Lower the body no further than legs parallel to the floor.

    An easy way to check for proper weight distribution is to try wiggling your toes. If you can't wiggle them, then your weight is too far forward.

7. The upward phase is simply standing up while pushing through your heels.

8. Remember, keep the:

- Knees aligned over the toes.
- Back straight.
- Weight on heels.

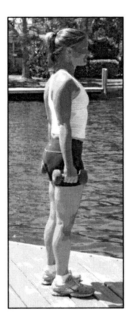 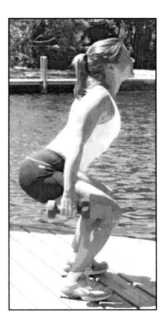

Scuba Application

This will allow you to rise from a bench in full gear with less effort. It will also make climbing that ladder after your dive easier.

Hint

Yet another easy activity to squeeze in at the office…just be sure that nobody is watching you.

STATIONARY LUNGE

The lunge is another exercise for the lower body. It is good for strengthening in addition to maintaining your range of motion.

Setup

Stand with your feet shoulder width apart. Maintain an athletic stance with shoulders and buttocks back.

Exercise

1. Take a step backwards with your right foot.

2. The left knee should be over the left heel.

3. Lower the right knee to floor.

4. Remember to maintain a straight back.

5. Just before the right knee touches the ground, stand, returning to the starting position.

6. Bring your feet together for starting position.

7. Repeat the same routine with the left foot back.

8. That is one rep.

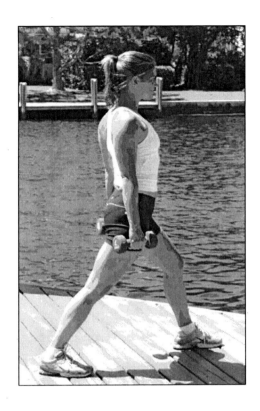 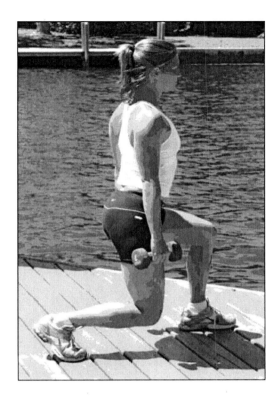

Scuba Application

This will allow you to rise from a bench in full gear with less effort. It will also make climbing the ladder and walking around in full gear easier.

Tip

Make sure that your front knee does not pass your toe.

STANDING CALF RAISE

This exercise will strengthen your calves.

Setup

This will be done in a standing position using an ordinary household step. Stand with your heels hanging over the edge of a step. Use a wall or railing for balance.

Exercise

1. Stand up on the balls of your feet.

2. Hold for a count of two.

3. Slowly return to the starting position.

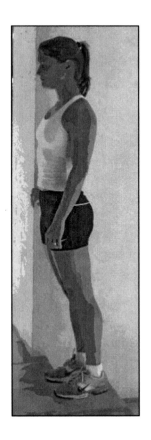 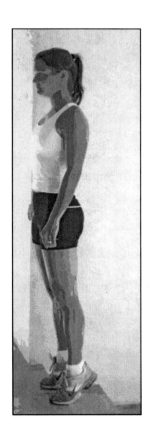

Scuba Application

This will make walking down the sand for those beach dives easier.

Hint

Calf raises can be done while standing in an elevator or waiting for a friend. Fortunately, these exercises are quite easy to integrate into your day.

STABILITY BALL LEG CURL

This exercise is great for strengthening the hamstrings and gluteus.

Setup

Begin by lying flat on your back. Legs are fully extended with the heels on the ball. The arms should be at your sides for support.

Exercise

1. Lift the pelvis off the floor, while maintaining a flat back in the bridge position.

2. Flex the knee and bring the heels to the buttocks.

3. Extend the legs to the starting position.

4. Maintain the bridge position.

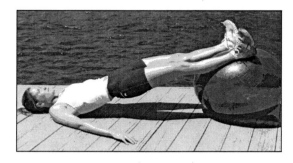 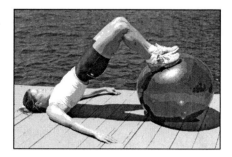

Scuba Application

This will make climbing down the ladder with gear on easier as well as returning to the bench to take off gear.

CHAPTER 7

Lower Body Gym

Exercise	Muscles	Scuba Applications
Smith Squat	Quadriceps Gluteus Hip Flexors	• Rising from bench • Sitting on bench • Walking in gear • Walking in sand • Setting gear on bench • Finning • Ascending/Descending ladder
Squat	Quadriceps Gluteus Hip Flexors	
Leg Press	Quadriceps Gluteus Hip Flexors	
Leg Extension	Quadriceps	
Leg Curl	Hamstrings Gastrocnemius	
Straight Leg Calf Raise	Gastrocnemius Soleus	

Hint

These workouts are awesome because when you walk into the gym, you are mentally prepared for your workout. Here, you will definitely work up a sweat.

SMITH SQUAT

This is a good transition from the body squat to a free weight squat. The machine will guide the weight and aid in your alignment.

Setup

Grip the bar at shoulder width. Step under the bar, allowing it to rest on your upper back. Straighten your knees to release the bar from the safety. Twist the bar free from the safety.

Exercise

1. Bend the knees, allowing the hips to move toward the floor.

2. Maintain a flat and rigid back.

3. Look forward with the chest out.

4. Knees should be aligned over the feet.

5. Don't let the knees go over the toes.

6. Lower the weight no further than thighs parallel to the floor.

*An easy way to check for proper weight distribution is the ability to wiggle your toes. If you can't wiggle them, then your weight is too far forward.

7. The upward phase is simply standing up.

8. Push up through the heels to the starting position.

9. Remember:

   - Do not let knees go past toes.
   - Shoulders and buttocks are back.
   - Weight is on heels.

10. After completing the set, re-rack the weight carefully.

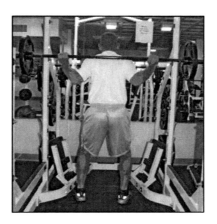

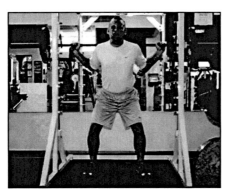 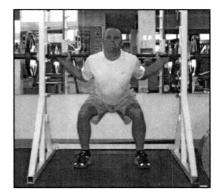

Scuba Application

The squat movements will help to strengthen the muscles needed for rising from a bench and climbing a ladder with your gear. As you know, all that gear adds a considerable amount of weight. The hips are also activated in the squat, which will improve your finning performance.

SQUAT

Simply squat from the standing position by bending the knees and lowering the hips to the floor. Having a spotter present is beneficial for safety.

Setup

Grip the bar at shoulder width. Step under the bar, allowing it to rest on the upper back. Stand up under the bar, releasing from the rack. Take a step backward to free of any obstruction. In standing position, the feet should be slightly wider than shoulder width apart with the toes pointed slightly outward. The back should always be flat. Push your rear out, shoulders back, and chest out.

Exercise

1. Bend the knees, allowing the hips to move toward the floor.

2. Maintain a flat and rigid back.

3. Look forward with the chest out.

4. Knees should be aligned over the feet.

5. Don't let the knees go over the toes.

6. Lower your body no further than thighs parallel to the floor.

7. The upward phase is simply standing up.

8. Push up through the heels to the starting position.

9. Remember:

- Do not let knees go past toes.

- Shoulders and buttocks are back.

- Weight is on heels.

10. After completing the set, re-rack the weight carefully.

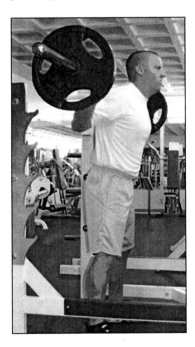 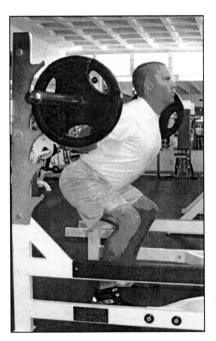

Scuba Application

The squat movements will help to strengthen the muscles needed for rising from a bench and climbing a ladder with your gear. As you know, all that gear adds a considerable amount of weight. The hips are also activated in the squat, which will improve your finning performance.

LEG PRESS

The leg press is similar to the squat, but it is done on a machine. The machine aids in guiding the movement of the weight; therefore, a spotter is not necessary.

Setup

Sit on the machine and place your feet on the foot pad. The feet should be shoulder width apart with the toes slightly angled out. Keep back and rear flat against the back pad and seat.

Exercise

1. Press the weight away from your body in a controlled manner.

2. Lower the weight no further than thighs parallel to the foot pad.

3. Push the foot pad away until the legs are almost fully extended.

4. Repeat the movement until all repetitions are complete.

5. Once the exercise is complete, make sure to replace the safety devices before releasing the weight.

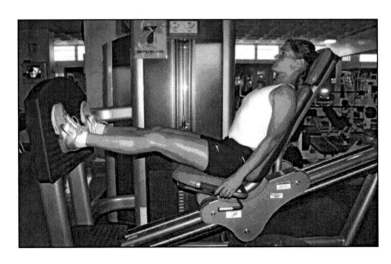

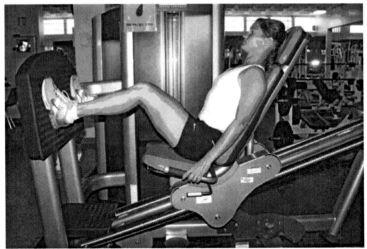

Scuba Application

The leg press will help to strengthen the muscles needed for rising from a bench and climbing a ladder with your gear. As you know, all that gear adds a considerable amount of weight.

LEG EXTENSION

This exercise consists of sitting in a fixed position and extending the legs at the knee. Proper body position in relation to the machine is key.

Setup

Adjust the backrest so that when you sit on the machine your knee is directly in line with the pivot point of the machine. The leg pad of the machine will be on the front of the leg (shin) just above the shoes. Hands should be by your side; usually, there are handles. Once the machine is properly set up, the exercise is easy.

Exercise

1. Extend your legs until your knees are straight.

2. Hold for a count of two.

3. Bring the weight down to the starting position.

4. Just before the weight touches, repeat the exercise for the proper number of reps.

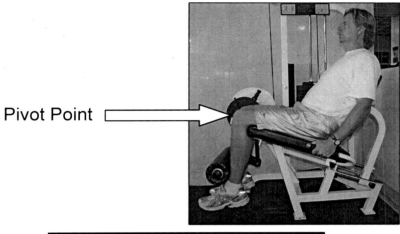

Pivot Point

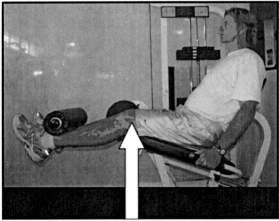

Pivot Point

Scuba Application

The leg extension will help to strengthen the muscles needed for rising from a bench and climbing a ladder with your gear. As you know, all that gear adds a considerable amount of weight.

LEG CURL

These are done lying on your stomach and bringing your heels to your buttocks by flexing the knees. This exercise is performed on a machine, so the setup and proper body position are important.

Setup

The only adjustment for this exercise is the leg pad, which should be just above the back of the shoe, when lying down. Lie on the machine with your feet under the leg pad. Hands should be placed on the handles under the stomach pad. Toes should be pointing to the floor.

Exercise

1. Bring your heels as close to your buttocks as you can without your pelvis coming off the pad.

2. The pad should be brought to your rear.

3. Lower the pad back to starting position.

4. Remember to repeat the exercise just before the weight touches the weight stack.

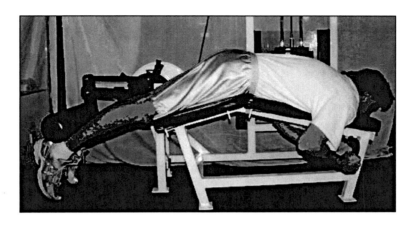

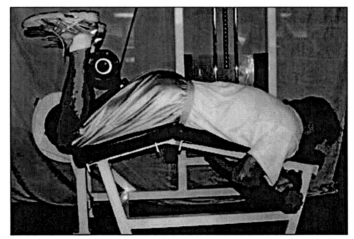

Scuba Application

When you are going down the ladder to begin your dive, your hamstrings help control you and all that extra weight. After completing your dive, you can confidently return to your seat to talk about the huge fish or amazing coral.

STRAIGHT LEG CALF RAISE

This exercise will strengthen your calf muscles.

Setup

Sit in the machine with the foot pad slightly closer than the length of your legs. Place feet shoulder width apart with only the balls of your feet on the pad. Maintain a slight bend in your knees.

Exercise

1. Point your toes, pushing the weight forward.

2. Slowly return to the starting position.

3. Repeat.

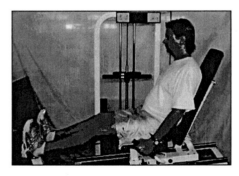 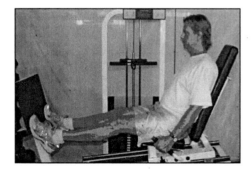

Scuba Application

You know the effect walking in the sand can have on your calves. The calf raise will allow you to plow through the sand to your dive entry with greater ease. Improving the strength of these muscles can also improve your finning performance.

CHAPTER 8

Upper Body Home Exercises

Exercise	Muscles	Scuba Applications
Pushup	Pectoralis Deltoids Triceps	• Climbing into inflatable boat • Climbing ladder • Lifting gear • Carrying tanks • Rising from bench
Shoulder Press	Deltoids	
Upright Row	Trapezius Deltoids	
Triceps Dip	Triceps Pectoralis	
Biceps Curl	Biceps Curl	
Bent Over Row	Latissimus Dorsi Trapezius Deltoids	
One Arm Row	Latissimus Dorsi Trapezius Deltoids	
Dumbbell Chest	Pectoralis	
Dumbbell Fly	Pectoralis	
Shoulder Raises	Deltoids	
Triceps Kickback	Triceps	

PUSHUP

Everyone already knows this one, but we will go over how to perform it correctly. As with every exercise, form is better than weight. We will progress from the knees to the toes.

Setup

Lie on the floor on your stomach. Place your hands under your shoulders with fingers pointing forward. The rest of the body should be nice and straight with the head in a neutral position. Looking down, your back and legs should remain in a straight line.

Exercise

1. Push up from the floor position by extending the arms.

2. Bend at the knees.

3. Fully extend the arms.

4. Lower your chest to the floor.

5. Touch the floor for just a second and push up again.

6. Repeat the required repetitions without stopping.

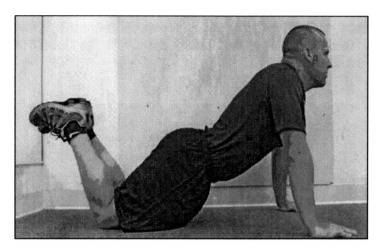

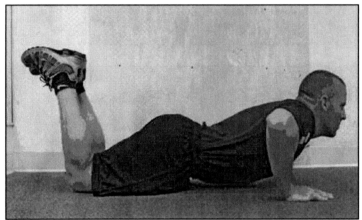

Tip

Keep your back flat.

Once you have mastered pushups on your knees, move on to the toe pushups. Everything is the same, but we are now using our toes as the contact point with the floor. Maintain a nice straight line from the toes to the head.

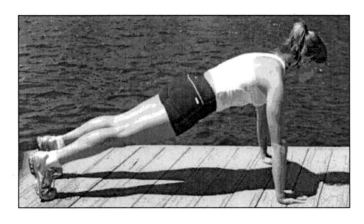

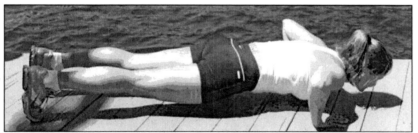

Scuba Application

Diving out of an inflatable boat is always fun. Getting dropped off at the dive site and picked up is great until it is time to get back in. Pushups will help you climb over the edge of the inflatable with greater ease. You will have a stronger push to lift your body those final inches from the water.

PHYSIO-BALL PUSHUP

This is a variation of the traditional pushup. Exercise difficulty can be decreased or increased with the use of the ball. Placing the ball under your hips or thighs actually makes the pushups easier. As the ball is rolled closer to the toes, the challenge also increases. One of the most challenging exercises is actually performing the pushup on the ball. The ball activates the abdominals more than the traditional pushup.

Setup

Regardless of the type of pushup, maintain a flat back. You can start with the ball under your hips and gradually roll it back to the toes.

Exercise

1. Bend your elbows so that your chest is about 1 inch from the floor or ball.

2. Press to the starting position.

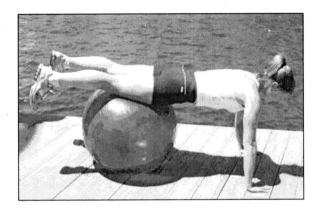 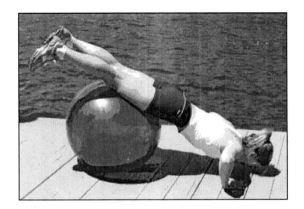

Try challenging yourself by rolling out further on the physio-ball. This will increase the use of your stabilization muscles, including your abdominals and lower back.

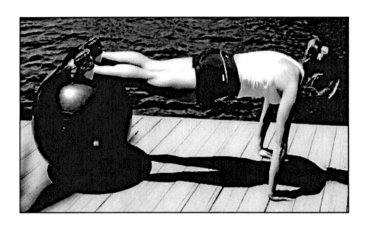

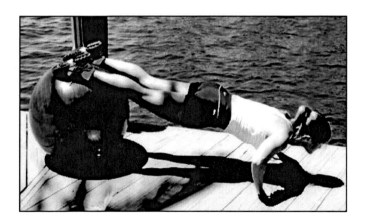

Now try the opposite starting position. Place your hands on the physio-ball and your toes on the ground. Make sure that your fingers point outwards, so that your weight does not roll the ball forward (causing you to do a faceplant on the ground).

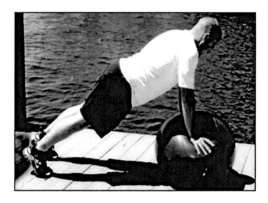

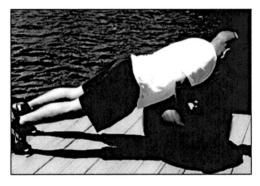

Scuba Application

Diving out of an inflatable boat is always fun. Getting dropped off at the dive site and picked up is great until it is time to get back in. Pushups will help you climb over the edge of the inflatable with greater ease. You will have a stronger push to lift your body those final inches from the water.

SHOULDER PRESS

This is done in the seated position while pushing a weight overhead. Any sturdy chair can be used for this exercise. Preferably not the couch or La-Z-Boy; they aren't highly motivational.

Setup

Sit up straight with both feet flat on the floor.

Exercise

1. Place a dumbbell in each hand.

2. Bring the weights to shoulder level.

3. Push the weight straight up overhead.

4. Fully extend the arms.

5. Slowly lower the weight to ear level.

6. Repeat for the proper number of sets.

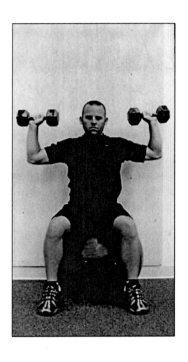 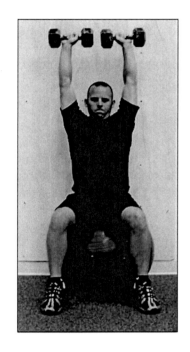

Scuba Application

The shoulders are involved in a number of lifting activities such as lifting equipment and entering an inflatable from the water.

UPRIGHT ROW

Upright rows are done in the standing position with resistance. The resistance can be dumbbells or a barbell.

Setup

Stand straight with your feet about shoulder width apart, forming a strong base. The dumbbells will begin at waist level with arms fully extended.

Exercise

1. Pull the dumbbells in a straight line toward the chin.

2. Maintain a straight back.

3. The elbows should be higher than the weights.

4. Slowly lower the weight once it has reached just below the shoulder.

5. Lower the weight to the starting position.

Key Points: Always maintain an athletic stance and execute movements in a controlled manner.

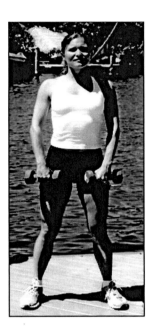 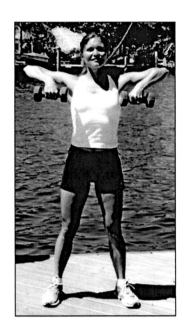

Scuba Application

Just looking at this picture makes you think of lifting a heavy bag of equipment or a tank onto the boat.

TRICEPS DIP

Dips can be done on a sturdy chair or bench.

Setup

Place your hands on the edge of the chair or bench. Place your feet out in front on the floor.

Exercise

1. Bend your elbows, no further than 90 degrees.

2. Allow the body to travel in a straight line toward the floor.

3. Push up to return to the starting position.

Tip

Only descend as low as you feel comfortable.

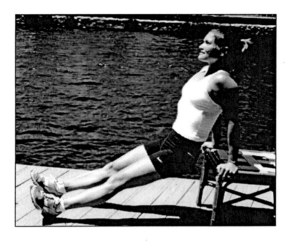

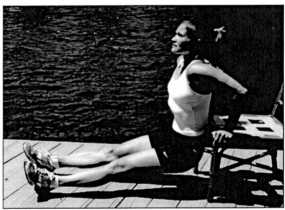

Scuba Application

A little help from your arms when getting up from a bench while loaded with gear is always an added benefit.

BICEPS CURL

This is where you get those guns you have always wanted. Concentrate on proper form to really isolate the biceps.

Setup

Begin in the seated position. Sit up straight with your arms at your sides. The shoulders and back should remain stationary to isolate the bicep. Your elbow should be directly at the side and remain stationary.

Exercise

1. Raise one hand, palm facing up.

2. Bring the weight as far up as possible.

3. Slowly lower the weight to the starting position.

4. Perform the same motion with the other arm.

5. That is one repetition.

Remember: The shoulder, elbow and back should remain stationary. The movement is at the elbow, and this will give you the guns you have always wanted.

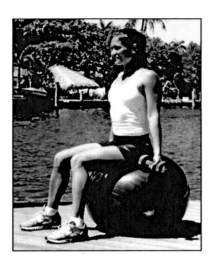 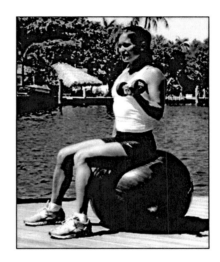

Scuba Application

Biceps strength is a bonus when pulling yourself up a ladder. These muscles also look great on the beach.

BENT OVER ROW

Proper body position is important to take the pressure off the back. Always maintain a rigid flat back throughout the exercise. Engage the abs to protect the lower back. This exercise will really work the muscles of the back.

Setup

Begin with a nice base; your feet should be slightly wider than shoulder width. There should be a bend at your knees and waist, allowing your upper body to move over your feet. Your back must remain flat throughout the exercise. Your hands will be directly below your chest with the weight.

Exercise

1. Pull the weight to your chest.

2. Hold for a two count.

3. Slowly lower the weight to the starting position.

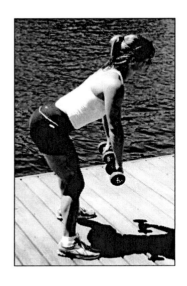 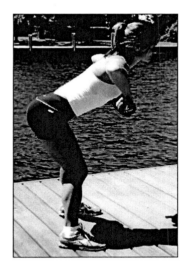

Scuba Application

This exercise will also allow you to pull yourself up the ladder much easier.

Tip

Look straight ahead.

ONE ARM ROW

This exercise uses more stabilizing muscles than the bent over row.

Setup

Begin in the same position as the bent over row. However, you may use a chair for support and your head should also maintain a neutral position. Also, your arm should hang naturally from your shoulder with your palm facing your body.

Exercise

1. Pull the weight to the chest.

2. Hold for a two count.

3. Slowly lower the weight to the starting position.

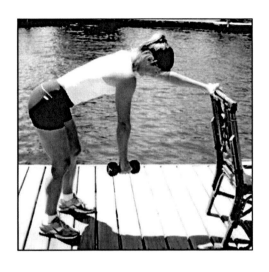 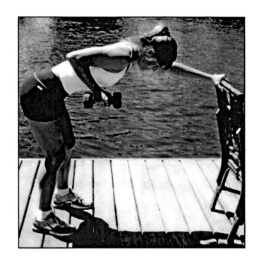

Scuba Application

This is a variation of the bent over row also allowing you to pull yourself up the ladder.

Tip

Look toward the ground.

DUMBBELL CHEST PRESS

This is a great dumbbell exercise for the chest.

Setup

Lie with your back supported by the ball. The dumbbells will be at chest level like the bottom of a bench press. While learning the exercise, start with lightweight dumbbells and progress with proper performance. Perfect form will yield the best results.

Exercise

1. Press the weights straight up.

2. Fully extend the elbows.

3. Repeat for the number of reps.

*Have a spotter, who will spot at the wrists. The spotter can also take the weights after completing the exercise. Make sure the weights are picked up away from the face.

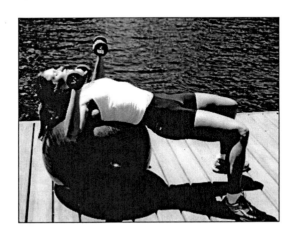 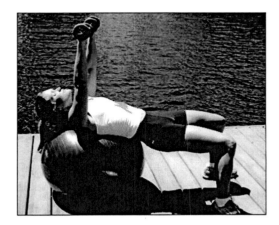

<u>*Scuba Application*</u>

The chest press is similar to the pushup, allowing you to climb over the edge of the inflatable with greater ease. You will have a stronger push to lift your body those final inches from the water.

DUMBBELL FLY

This is a great dumbbell exercise for the chest. It is done while lying on your back on the ball or a flat bench. While learning the exercise, use very light dumbbells and progress with proper performance.

Setup

Lie with your upper back supported with the ball. Begin with the dumbbells in the press position, extended above the chest.

Exercise

1. Palms should be facing each other.

2. Slightly bend your elbows while lowering the weights toward the floor.

3. Lower the dumbbells to eye level/bench level.

4. Maintain a slight bend in the elbows.

5. Bring the weight back to the starting position.

6. Palms are facing each other.

7. Don't bang the weight (this shows control).

8. Repeat for the proper number of reps.

9. Bring the weights to the chest.

10. Sit up.

* Have a spotter, who will spot at the wrists. The spotter can also take the weights after completing the exercise. Make sure weights are picked up away from the face.

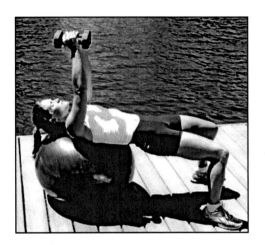 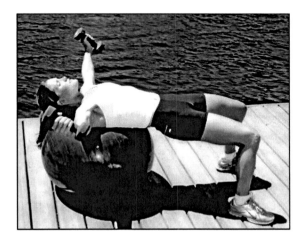

Scuba Application

Dumbbell flies will increase your chest musculature, which will balance out all the hard work you have done on your back. An imbalance of musculature may lead to injuries. Performing the fly exercise on the physio-ball incorporates additional muscles, such as the lower back and the abdominals, which stabilize the body.

FRONT SHOULDER RAISES

Shoulder raises will increase strength in the shoulders, which will decrease injury.

Setup

Begin in the athletic stance. Use light dumbbells with your hands at your sides with palms facing back for the front raises. Arms should be fully extended throughout the exercise.

Exercise

1. Raise the dumbbells directly in front one at time.

2. Stop at shoulder level.

3. Slowly lower the weight to the starting position.

4. Repeat the movement with the other hand.

*Maintain a rigid body throughout the exercise to focus on the shoulders.

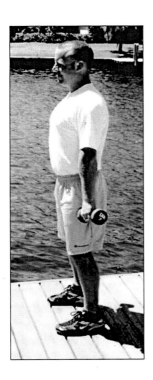 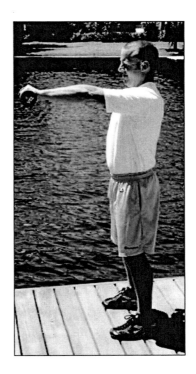

Scuba Application

The shoulders are involved in a number of lifting activities such as lifting equipment and entering an inflatable from the water.

LATERAL SHOULDER RAISES

Lateral shoulder raises are another exercise to strengthen the shoulders.

Setup

Begin with the athletic stance. Arms should be extended at your sides with. Your arms should be extended throughout the exercise with the palms facing down.

Exercise

1. Raise both dumbbells to shoulder height.

2. Slowly lower to the starting position.

3. Repeat.

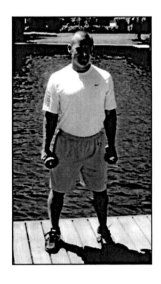 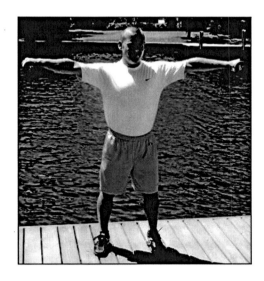

Scuba Application

The shoulders are involved in a number of lifting activities such as lifting equipment and entering an inflatable from the water.

TRICEPS KICKBACK

This exercise will strengthen your triceps.

Setup

Your feet should be shoulder width apart with your knees slightly bent. Bend at your hips so that your back is almost parallel to the ground. Raise your elbow posteriorly so that the top of your arm is parallel to the floor with the dumbbell in your hand. Your elbow should be close to your body and stationary. You may use a chair or bench for support as shown.

Exercise

1. Extend your dumbbell backwards at the elbow. (The movement is only at the elbow joint.)

2. Hold for a two-second count.

3. Slowly return to the starting position in a controlled manner.

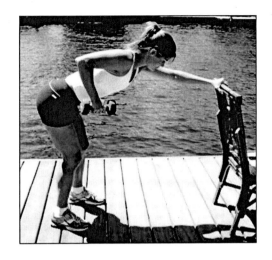 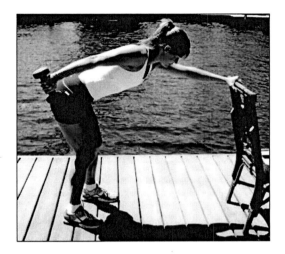

Scuba Application

A little help from your arms when getting up from a bench while loaded with gear is always an added benefit.

CHAPTER 9

Upper Body Gym Exercises

Exercise	Muscles	Scuba Applications
Bench Press	Pectoralis Deltoids Triceps	• Climbing into inflatable boat • Climbing ladder • Lifting gear • Carrying tanks • Rising from bench
Pec Deck Fly	Pectoralis	
Lat Pull Down	Latissimus Dorsi Biceps	
Military Press	Deltoids Triceps	
Seated Row	Latissimus Dorsi Trapezius Deltoids	
Triceps Push Down	Triceps	
Dip	Pectoralis Triceps	
Preacher Curl	Biceps	

BENCH PRESS

This exercise can be done with free weights or various machines. Once you have mastered this, the machines will be easy. This exercise is done while lying on your back on a bench and pressing a bar from the chest. Proper progression is very important to properly perform this exercise. This is an excellent upper body exercise when performed correctly.

Setup

Lie on the bench with your feet flat on the ground. You should not be able to look straight up at the bar on the rack. Slide down the bench so that you have to look back at the bar. Reach up and grip the bar with your hands slightly wider than shoulder width. Make sure they are even on the bar, by using the rough and smooth areas of the bar as references. Grip the rough surface; that is what it is for. Now you are properly set up.

* Most barbells weigh 45 lbs; try lighter barbells first if you are unsure if you are able to move this weight.

Exercise

1. Lift the bar off the rack (a spotter can help with this).

2. Position the bar just above the chest with arms fully extended.

3. Slowly and smoothly lower the bar to the chest (nipple line).

4. Lightly touch the chest (don't drop onto chest).

5. Press the bar from the chest to the starting position.

6. Extend arms fully.

7. Continue until proper number of reps are complete.

8. Re-rack the bar with the assistance of a spotter.

*A spotter should always be used when performing this exercise.

Remember five points of contact: Both Feet, Buttocks, Back, and Head.

DO NOT

Arch back.

Lift feet off floor or head off bench.

Use too much weight.

Bounce weight off chest.

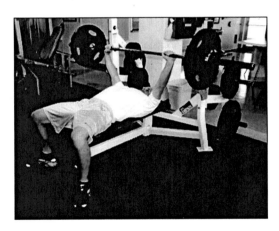 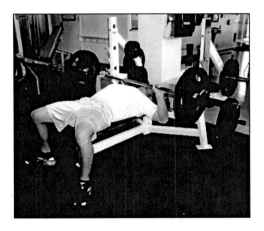

Scuba Application

Diving out of an inflatable boat is always fun. Getting dropped off at the dive site and picked up is great until it is time to get back in. Bench presses will help you climb over the edge of the inflatable with greater ease. You will have a stronger push to lift your body those final inches from the water.

PEC DECK FLY

This is another exercise for your chest. The machine will guide you, provided you have set it up properly.

Setup

Elevate the seat so that when you grasp the handles your arms are parallel to the floor. You will also need to set the end point range of motion. This will limit how far back you will have to go. Be conservative to start out, especially if shoulders are inflexible.

Exercise

1. Grasp the handles so that your arms are comfortably out at your sides.

2. Bring the handles in so that they meet in front of you.

3. Slowly return to the starting position in a controlled manner.

* As in all exercises, try not to rest the weights in between exercises.

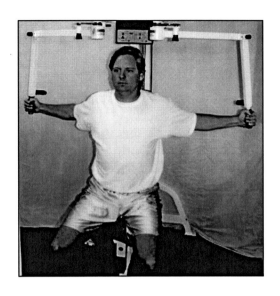 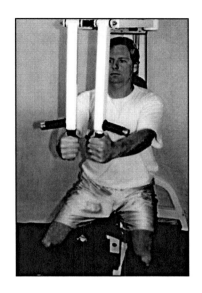

Scuba Application

Dumbbell flies will increase your chest musculature, which will balance out all the hard work you have done on your back. An imbalance of musculature may lead to injuries.

LAT PULL DOWN

Pulling exercises such as a lat pull down and a row will work the opposing muscles of the presses. Performing the lat pull down is done by pulling a bar connected to a weight to the upper chest while seated.

Setup

The seat and leg pad must be adjusted before beginning. While seated, the leg pad should rest on the thighs above the knee. The feet should be flat on the floor. During the exercise the back must remain rigid, since there is no back support. After the seat is adjusted, stand and grip the bar. The grip needs to be wider than shoulder width, usually at the bend in the bar.

Exercise

1. Grip bar evenly.

2. Sit on the seat with legs under the pad (this holds you down).

3. Keep the back straight and bend slightly at the hips, away from the machine.

4. Maintain this position.

5. Pull the bar to the upper chest just below the clavicles.

6. Slowly return the bar to the beginning position.

7. Don't let the weight pull you up, keep rear on seat.

8. Continue until all reps are completed.

9. Stand up while holding the bar, allow the weights to rest on the weight stack.

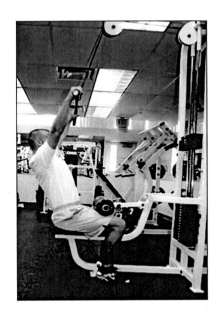 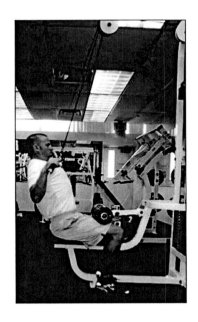

Scuba Application

This exercise will also allow you to pull yourself up the ladder much easier. The biceps will also be activated in the lat pull down.

MILITARY PRESS

This is done in a seated position on a machine while pushing a weight overhead. As with all the machines, setup is crucial for proper execution.

Setup

Adjust the seat so that the handles are just below ear level. The back and head should be flat against the back pad. Both feet need to be flat on the floor. For our purposes, grip the handles in the most comfortable position. Different positions target different areas of the shoulders.

Exercise

1. Push the weight overhead.

2. Fully extend the arms.

3. Lower the weight to ear level.

4. The weight should not touch the stack if the machine is properly set up.

5. Repeat for the proper number of sets.

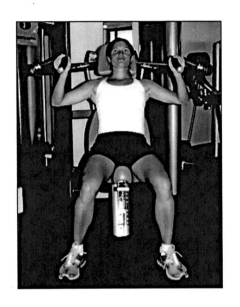 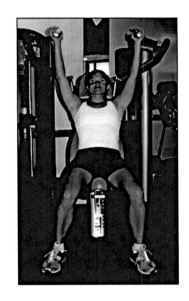

Scuba Application

The shoulders are involved in a number of lifting activities such as lifting equipment and entering an inflatable from the water.

SEATED ROW

A seated position with the feet extended and supported on a platform while pulling a bar toward you. There are no machine adjustments for this exercise.

Setup

From the seated position, the feet will be flat against the platform. The legs will remain stationary with the knees slightly bent. The bar, used for the row, positions the hands to be palm to palm. Make sure the back and the legs make a 90° angle. Bend at the knees to grip the bar, and then extend the legs to the starting position.

Exercise

1. Pull the bar toward your body just below the chest.

2. Keep the elbows close to the body.

3. Slowly extend arms away from the body.

4. Continue until all reps are completed.

5. Once all reps are completed, bend at your legs to lower the weight to the weight stack.

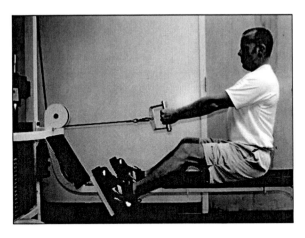

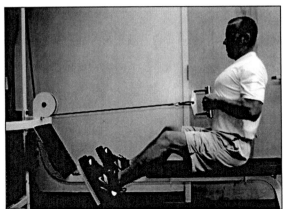

Scuba Application

This exercise will also allow you to easily pull yourself up the ladder.

TRICEPS PUSH DOWN

This exercise on the cable machine will strengthen your triceps.

Setup

As in all exercises, maintain an athletic stance. Your elbows should be at your sides, at an approximately 90° angle (imagine a rope tied around your waist and upper arms).

Exercise

1. Fully extend your elbows, pushing the bar toward the floor.

2. Slowly return to the starting position in a controlled manner.

*Make sure that the movement only occurs at your elbow. Many people have a tendency to move at the shoulder.

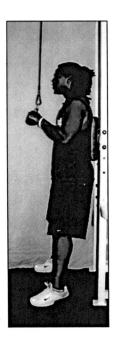 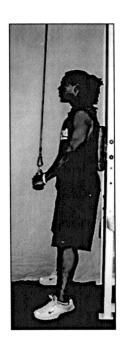

Scuba Application

A little help from your arms when getting up from a bench while loaded with gear is always an added benefit.

DIP

This exercise works your triceps as well as your chest. It is beneficial to integrate this exercise after you have mastered the triceps push down and the bench press.

Setup

Start with your hands on the bars and bend your knees so that they are clear of the floor.

Exercise

1. Straighten your elbows so that your arms are fully extended.

2. Slowly lower your body so that your elbow is at a 90° angle or greater.

* As you progress, you will be able to lower your body more and more.

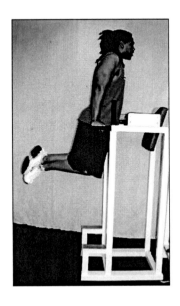 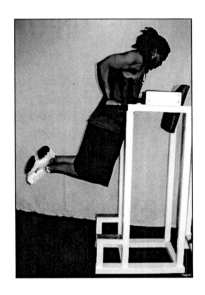

Scuba Application

A little help from your arms when getting up from a bench while loaded with gear is always an added benefit.

PREACHER CURL

This is a great exercise to isolate the biceps.

Setup

The pad should be adjusted so it comes just below the armpit. The back of your arms will be on the pad throughout the exercise. The weight will have to be taken off the rack; a partner is good for this.

Exercise

1. Begin with the arms fully extended with palms up.

2. Curl the bar up by flexing the arms.

3. Slowly lower the weight to the starting position.

* Do not use your shoulders or back; this will take the emphasis off the biceps.

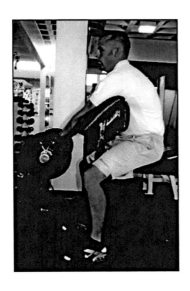 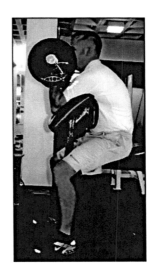

Scuba Application

Biceps strength is a bonus when pulling yourself up a ladder. These muscles also look good on the beach.

CHAPTER 10

Abdominal Exercises

Exercise	Muscles	Scuba Applications
Back Press	Rectus Abdominis	
Crunch	Rectus Abdominis	• Stability with gear on
Cross Crunch	Rectus Abdominis Obliques	• Balance on the boat
Ball Crunch	Rectus Abdominis	

Scuba Application

You have probably already experienced the shift in your center of gravity as soon as you don your gear. Increased abdominal strength will make all of the activities related to your dive easier. These core muscles are responsible for stability and balance. This is of particular importance when wearing heavy dive gear.

Hint

There is plenty of time to squeeze in sets of abdominal exercises during the commercial breaks of your favorite television shows.

BACK PRESS

This is a good starting point to establish proper form for abdominal exercises.

Setup

Begin by lying on your back on the floor with your knees bent.

Exercise

1. Press the lower back to the floor.

2. Contract the abdominal muscles.

3. Hold for a count of two seconds.

4. Return to the starting position.

5. Continue contracting and relaxing.

Lie on floor

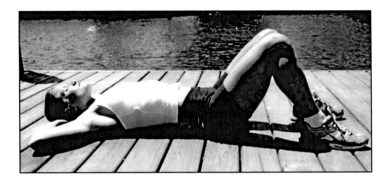

Press back to floor

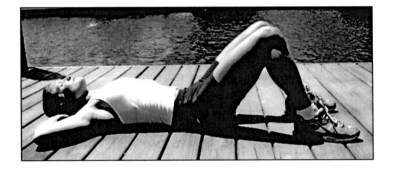

Hint

Take some time periodically throughout your day to tighten your abdominals. This can be accomplished by pulling your belly button in toward your spine. Try holding it for two, then five, then 30 seconds. This works quite well when you are sitting at your desk or in traffic, for those of us who have little free time to spare.

CRUNCH

This exercise is famous for building abdominals. Done *properly*, crunches can be very effective. Make sure to really concentrate on pressing your back to the floor.

Setup

Lie flat on the floor or mat with the knees bent. Use your abdominals to lift your shoulder blades off the floor while pressing your lower back into the floor.

Exercise

1. Contract the abdominal muscles.

2. Lift the shoulder blades up from the floor.

3. Hold for a count of two.

4. The lower back should maintain contact with the floor at all times.

5. Lower the shoulder blades back to the starting position.

6. Think "Six Pack" and continue.

* Make sure to master the previous exercises before moving on to more challenging exercises.

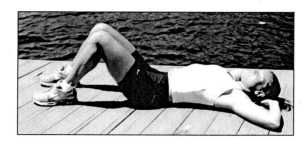 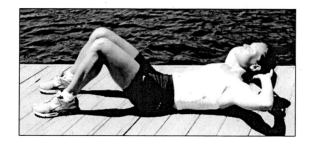

Variations: Once you have mastered the basic abdominal exercises, you can increase the lever arm to increase the difficulty of the exercise. Holding the hands extended over the head makes for an even more challenging crunch. Make sure to focus on form; don't swing the arms—this creates momentum and decreases the effectiveness of the exercise.

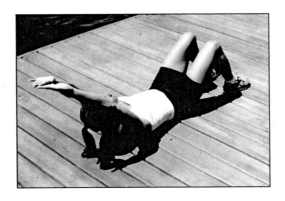

Add a medicine ball to further increase resistance.

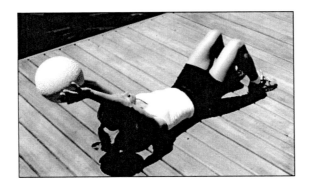

CROSS CRUNCH

These will add a little twist to the ordinary crunch. This twist stimulates the obliques.

Setup

Lie on the floor with one knee bent and the other crossed. Place one hand behind your head and the other at your side.

Exercise

1. Lift the right elbow and touch the left knee.

2. Hold for two seconds.

3. Return to the starting position.

4. Take the left elbow and touch the right knee.

5. That is one repetition.

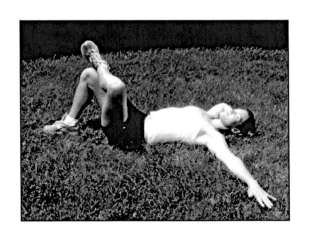

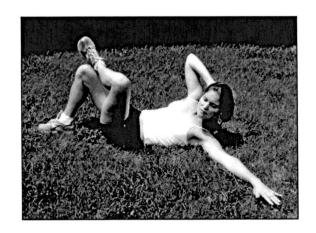

107

BALL CRUNCH

A ball can be used to add some variation to the workout. This increases recruitment of stabilizing muscles.

Setup

Lie with entire upper back supported by the ball. Place feet flat on the floor with the knees at a 90-degree angle. The arms may be behind the head. Remember not to pull up on the head. The back should be in a straight line.

Exercise

1. Raise the chest up to the sky using your abdominals.

2. Hold the contraction for two seconds.

3. Slowly lower the upper body to the starting position.

4. Maintain the abdominal contraction throughout the movement.

5. Continue until the sets are completed.

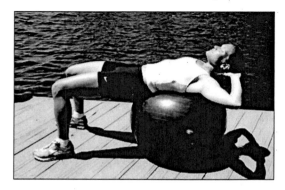 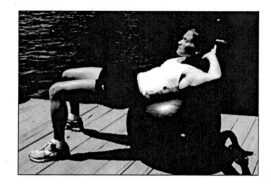

Variations: Increasing the lever arm adds resistance, similar to the crunch.

1. Place the arms overhead.

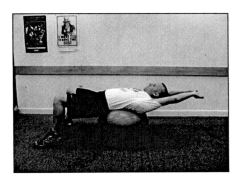 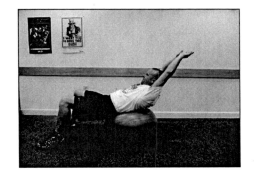

2. Hold a light ball at the chest.

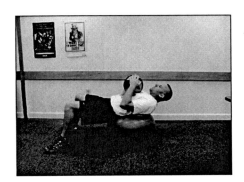 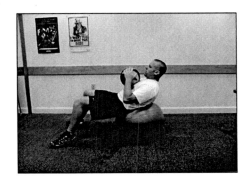

3. Hold a light ball overhead.

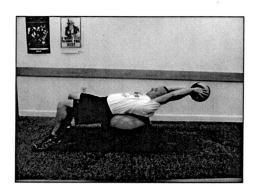 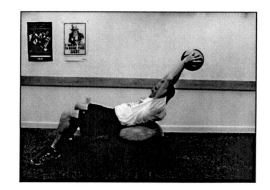

4. Cross Crunch.

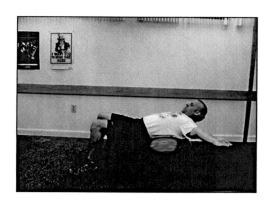 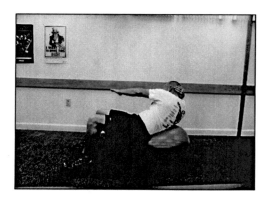

CHAPTER 11

Lower Back Exercises

Exercise	Muscles	Scuba Applications
Arm and Leg Raise	Erector Spinae	• Finning
Quadruped	Erector Spinae	• Stability with gear on
Back Extension	Erector Spinae	• Reduced lower back pain
Roman Chair	Erector Spinae	

SCUBA APPLICATION

Increased strength in your lower back is important for balancing all of the abdominal work that you have been doing. It will also help reduce or prevent lower back pain if performed regularly. A strong lower back will improve your finning capability as well as your overall stability.

ARM and LEG RAISE

This is a simple exercise to build strength in the lower back.

Setup

Lie flat on the floor on your stomach. Extend the arms as if you were flying. It may be more comfortable to use a mat.

Exercise

1. Simultaneously, raise opposite hand and opposite foot off the floor.

2. Then try simultaneously, raising your hands and feet off the floor.

3. Hold for a count of two.

4. Slowly lower yourself back to starting position.

5. That's one repetition.

6. Continue until all reps are complete.

* As you progress, increase holding time and height slightly.

Starting Position

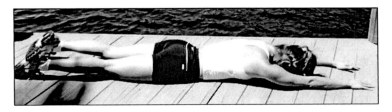

Alternate Raises

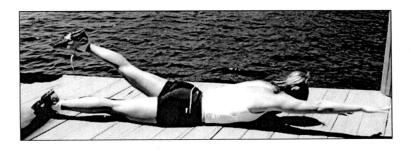

Superman

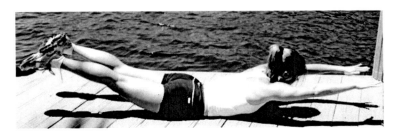

QUADRUPED

This exercise focuses on strengthening the lower back while improving your sense of balance.

Setup

Start with your hands and knees on the floor. Maintain a flat back and neutral head position.

Exercise

1. Raise your right hand and left leg.

2. Reach out with your fingers and toes.

3. There should be a straight line from your fingers to the toes.

4. Hold for two seconds.

5. Lower your hand and foot back to starting position.

6. Raise your left hand and right leg.

7. Hold for two seconds.

8. Return to starting position.

9. That is one repetition.

* For more of a challenge, raise the same leg and arm. This will really challenge your sense of balance.

Starting Position

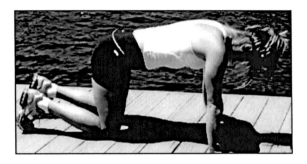

Alternate Raises

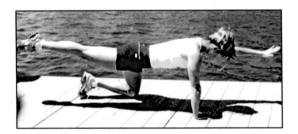

Same Side Raises

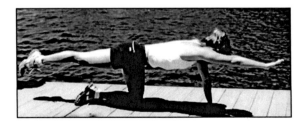

BACK EXTENSION

This exercise will improve lower back strength in addition to balance.

Setup

Lie on the ball with feet slightly wider than shoulder width and hands behind the head. The wider the stance, the easier it is to balance.

Exercise

1. Raise your head and shoulders up until you have a straight back.

2. Lower your body slowly.

3. Repeat.

* To increase resistance, increase the lever arm as in sit-ups.

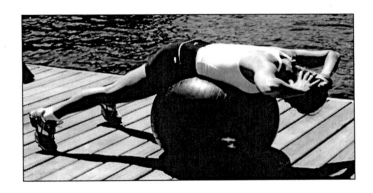

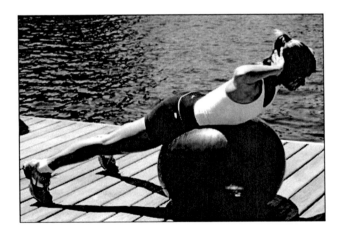

ROMAN CHAIR

There is no sitting in the roman chair. For this exercise, your legs will be held stationary while bending at the waist. This will improve your lower back strength.

Setup

The roman chair may or may not be adjustable. Typically the thighs will rest on a pad and the back of the heels will be under a pad. Your legs will be stationary, allowing the upper body to move. Maintain a flat rigid back throughout the exercise. Rest your hands behind your head.

Exercise

1. Bend at the waist allowing the head to move toward the floor.

2. Stop momentum for a one count.

3. Return the upper body to the starting position slowly.

4. Do not hyperextend the back or go past its normal position.

5. Continue this smooth movement until all reps are complete.

* To increase resistance, try holding a weight against your chest.

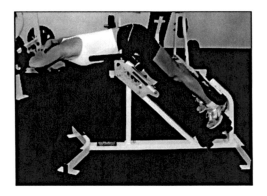

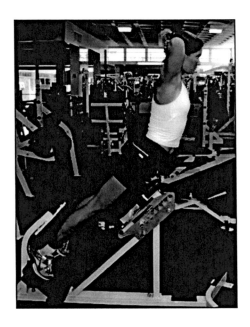

CHAPTER 12

Cardiovascular Exercises

Cardiovascular exercises will improve the efficiency of your oxygen usage. This may decrease your breathing frequency while increasing your bottom time within the limits of your dive plan. It will also make long swims and challenging currents less stressful, increasing the enjoyment of your dive.

A good starting point for cardiovascular exercise is an accumulation of 30 minutes of aerobic activity per day. Gradually increase the duration of each cardiovascular session until you can complete at least 30 minutes of continuous aerobic activity. Once you have reached this point, it is time to increase the intensity of your cardiovascular workout.

You may participate in any combination of aerobic activities to improve cardiovascular endurance. It doesn't matter which activity you choose, as long as you maintain an elevated heart rate for the duration of your workout.

Sample cardiovascular exercises include, but are not limited to, the following:

- Walking
- Jogging
- Swimming
- Cycling
- Stair climbing
- Cross-country skiing

Traditionally, three options are available to determine your level of exertion. The simplest evaluation is the talk test. A more specific estimate of cardiovascular exertion is the Rate of Perceived Exertion. The most specific field assessment of cardiovascular exertion is to use a target heart rate.

TALK TEST

The talk test is just as it sounds. During your exercise, try to talk. If you can hear your breathing, you are exercising at a moderate intensity. If you cannot talk, you are exercising vigorously.

Activity	Intensity
Able to sing	Light
Comfortable conversation	Moderate
Too out of breath to talk	Vigorous

Rate of Perceived Exertion

The rate of perceived exertion (RPE) is a simple scale from 1 to 10. It is beneficial to record your RPE for each cardiovascular activity in your exercise log.

Score	Exertion Level
1	No Exertion
2	Extremely Light
3	Fairly Light
4	Light
5	Moderate
6	Moderately Heavy
7	Fairly Heavy
8	Very Heavy
9	Extremely Heavy
10	Maximal Exertion

TARGET HEART RATE

The target heart rate is a direct measurement of cardiovascular exertion. You simply take your one-minute heart rate. For this evaluation, you may use a heart-rate monitor, carotid pulse, or radial pulse. Use two fingers as shown in the diagrams below to palpate your pulse. Do not use your thumb because it has a small pulse of its own. Your target range should be between 60% and 80% of your maximum heart rate. When you begin your programming, your goal should be closer to 60%. But as your fitness improves, your percentage should gradually increase.

Carotid Pulse

Radial Pulse

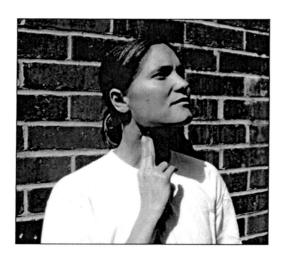
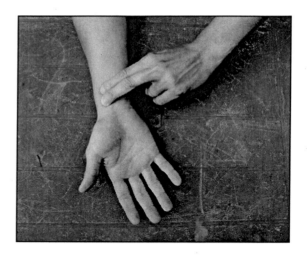

How to calculate your maximum heart rate:

$$220 - Age = Max\ Heart\ Rate$$

How to calculate your target heart rate range:

Moderate Intensity

Max Heart Rate X .50 = lower limit of range

Max Heart Rate X .70 = upper limit of range

Vigorous Intensity

Max Heart Rate X .60 = lower limit of range

Max Heart Rate X .80 = upper limit of range

Range:

Lower Limit – Upper Limit = Range of Beats

CHAPTER 13

Hydration

Proper hydration is vital to your safety and success! It is important to replace lost fluids. When you participate in an exercise program, you lose an increased amount of bodily fluids due to sweating. This fluid must be replaced via proper hydration. If you are ingesting fluids other than water, be aware of the calories associated with those fluids. Soft drinks and juices contain a high number of calories; sports drinks contain less calories, and water contains zero calories. This is of particular importance if weight loss is one of your goals.

Tips

- Always have water available; carry a water bottle to sip throughout the day.

- Don't wait until you are thirsty to drink.

- Drink eight ounces of water pre- and post-workout.

- Sip every 15 minutes throughout the workout and additionally as needed.

- Drinking water prior to each meal will help you stay full.

127

Nutrition

Proper nutrition is an integral component of a successful fitness program. A balanced moderate diet is the key to your success. Food is the source of energy for all of the functions of your body. Your body will run more efficiently with a complete balanced diet. Although we are not dieticians, we can offer a few tips.

Tips

- Only eat when you are hungry.

- Have larger meals earlier in the day.

- Even fat-free food sources are stored as body fat when they are not used.

- Choose complex carbohydrate sources, such as whole grain breads rather than white. They:

    o Provide an even energy source throughout the day.

    o Use more energy to break down.

    o Are usually more nutrient dense.

- Limit fat consumption to < 30% of total calories.

    o The # of calories from fat is provided on the food label.

- Limit saturated fats to < 10% of total calories.

    o Saturated fats are usually solid at room temperature.

    o Unsaturated fats are usually liquid at room temperature.

APPENDICES

EXERCISE LOG

DATE: _____   DAY: _____

EXERCISE	SET 1		SET 2		SET 3		COMMENTS
	W	R	W	R	W	R	

Weekly Goal:

SAMPLE WORKOUTS

3-Day Program

Home			
	Day 1	**Day 2**	**Day 3**
Weeks 1-2	Upper Body Sets: 1 Reps: 10	Lower Body Sets: 1 Reps: 10	Combo Sets: 1 Reps: 10
Weeks 3-4	Upper Body Sets: 2 Reps: 10-12	Lower Body Sets: 2 Reps: 10-12	Combo Sets: 2 Reps: 10-12
Weeks 5-8	Lower Body Sets: 3 Reps: 10-15	Lower Body Sets: 3 Reps: 10-15	Combo Sets: 3 Reps: 10-15

Upper Body	**Lower Body**	**Combo**
Pushup	Body/Chair Squat	Dumbbell Press/Fly
Upright Row	Standing Calf Raise	Bent One Arm Row
Shoulder Press	Back Press	Shoulder Raise
Bent Over Row	Back Extension	Triceps Dip/Kickback
Quadruped	Crunch	Biceps Curl
Back Press	Arm and Leg Raise	Stationary Lunge
Arm and Leg Raise	Cross Crunch	Stability Ball Leg Curl
Crunch		Ball Crunch

Gym			
	Day 1	**Day 2**	**Day 3**
Weeks 1-2	Upper Body Sets: 1 Reps: 10	Lower Body Sets: 1 Reps: 10	Combo Sets: 1 Reps: 10
Weeks 3-4	Upper Body Sets: 2 Reps: 10-12	Lower Body Sets: 2 Reps: 10-12	Combo Sets: 2 Reps: 10-12
Weeks 5-8	Lower Body Sets: 3 Reps: 10-15	Upper Body Sets: 3 Reps: 10-15	Combo Sets: 3 Reps: 10-15

Upper Body	**Lower Body**	**Combo**
Chest Press	Squat	Dip
Seated Row	Straight Leg Calf Raise	Lat Pull Down
Military Press	Leg Press	Pec Dec
Lat Pull Down	Back Press	Triceps Extension
Quadruped	Crunch	Preacher Curl
Back Press	Back Extension	Leg Extension
Arm and Leg Raise	Arm and Leg Raise	Leg Curl
Crunch	Cross Crunch	Roman Chair
		Crunch

4-Day Program

Home				
	Day 1	**Day 2**	**Day 3**	**Day 4**
Weeks 1-2	Upper Body Sets: 1 Reps: 10	Lower Body Sets: 1 Reps: 10	Upper Body Sets: 1 Reps: 10	Lower Body Sets: 1 Reps: 10
Weeks 3-4	Upper Body Sets: 2 Reps: 10-12	Lower Body Sets: 2 Reps: 10-12	Upper Body Sets: 2 Reps: 10-12	Lower Body Sets: 2 Reps: 10-12
Weeks 5-8	Lower Body Sets: 3 Reps: 10-15	Upper Body Sets: 3 Reps: 10-15	Lower Body Sets: 3 Reps: 10-15	Upper Body Sets: 3 Reps: 10-15

Upper Body	**Lower Body**	**Upper Body**	**Lower Body**
Push Up	Chair/Box Squat	Dumbbell Press or Fly	Body Squat
Bent Over Row	Stationary Lunge	Bent Over Row	Stationary Lunge
Military Press	Stability Ball Leg Curl	Shoulder Raise	Stability Ball Leg Curl
Bent Over Row	Standing Calf Raise	Biceps Curl	Standing Calf Raise
Triceps Dip	Roman Chair	Triceps Kickback	Roman Chair
Back Press	Ball Crunch	Back Extension	Ball Crunch
Leg/Arm Raise		Crunch	
Crunch			

Gym				
	Day 1	**Day 2**	**Day 3**	**Day 4**
Weeks 1-2	Upper Body Sets: 1 Reps: 10	Lower Body Sets: 1 Reps: 10	Upper Body Sets: 1 Reps: 10	Lower Body Sets: 1 Reps: 10
Weeks 3-4	Upper Body Sets: 2 Reps: 10-12	Lower Body Sets: 2 Reps: 10-12	Upper Body Sets: 2 Reps: 10-12	Lower Body Sets: 2 Reps: 10-12
Weeks 5-8	Lower Body Sets: 3 Reps: 10-15	Upper Body Sets: 3 Reps: 10-15	Lower Body Sets: 3 Reps: 10-15	Upper Body Sets: 3 Reps: 10-15

Upper Body	**Lower Body**	**Upper Body**	**Lower Body**
Chest Press	Squat	Pec Deck	Squat
Seated Row	Leg Press	Seated Row	Leg Press
Military Press	Leg Curl	Military Press	Leg Curl
Lat Pull Down	Leg Extension	Dip	Leg Extension
Triceps Push Down	Seated Calf Raise	Preacher Curl	Seated Calf Raise
Preacher Curl	Roman Chair	Triceps Push Down	Roman Chair
Leg/Arm Raise	Ball Crunch	Quadruped Crunch	Ball Crunch
Crunch			

CPSIA information can be obtained at www.ICGtesting.com
Printed in the USA
BVOW04s0814220915

419068BV00014B/2/P

9 780741 431110